GW01034069

Best Herbal Medicine and Healing Food From Nature to Prevent Insomnia Plus Make Sleep Better English Edition

Jannah Firdaus Mediapro

Published by Jannah Firdaus Mediapro Studio, 2021.

While every precaution has been taken in the preparation of this book, the publisher assumes no responsibility for errors or omissions, or for damages resulting from the use of the information contained herein.

BEST HERBAL MEDICINE AND HEALING FOOD FROM NATURE TO PREVENT INSOMNIA PLUS MAKE SLEEP BETTER ENGLISH EDITION

First edition. June 7, 2021.

Copyright © 2021 Jannah Firdaus Mediapro.

Written by Jannah Firdaus Mediapro.

Table of Contents

Prologue

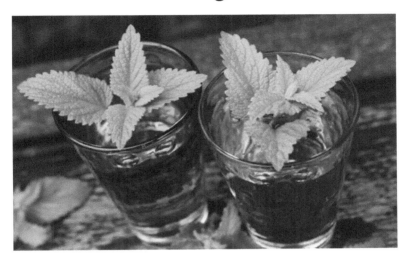

Insomnia is characterized by an inability to obtain a sufficient amount of sleep to feel rested. It can be due to either difficulty falling or staying asleep. It may also result in waking earlier than desired.

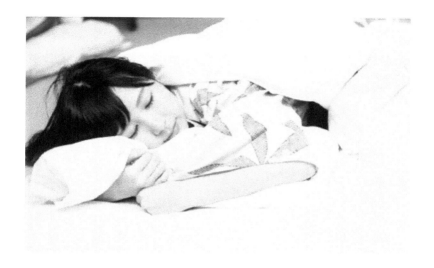

The sleep is often reported to be of chronically poor quality and light and unrefreshing. As a result of this, people with insomnia suffer from daytime symptoms like poor attention, irritability, and reduced energy.

Fortunately, there are effective treatment options for insomnia, ranging from the temporary use of sleeping pills, cognitive behavioral therapy and using herbal medicine treatment from nature.

1. Valerian Root

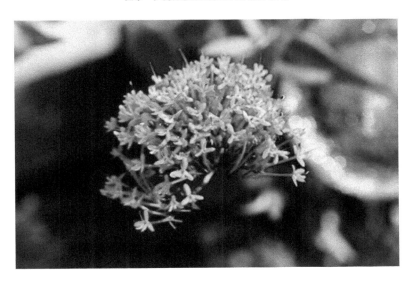

Valerian (Valeriana officinalis) is a herbal home remedy, brewed as a tea or taken as a supplement, that is commonly used to reduce anxiety, improve sleep quality, and act as a sedative. Clinical trials of valerian have had inconsistent results for insomnia.

Studies measuring sleep quality have found no difference between people taking valerian and those taking a placebo. However, a sizable number of people in the studies anecdotally reported that their sleep quality improved with valerian.

Valerian is thought to affect levels of one of the calming neurotransmitters in the body, gamma-aminobutyric acid (GABA). It also relieves muscle spasms and is thought to help alleviate menstrual period pain.

2. Lemon Balm

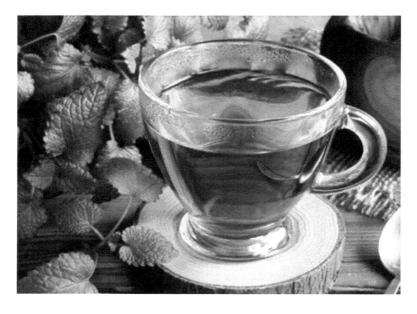

Melissa officinalis (Lemon balm) is a tea and herbal supplement that is said to relieve anxiety and calm the nerves. It may be seen in supplements that also include valerian.

Drink lemon balm tea at night to make sleep better and natural.

3. Chamomile Tea

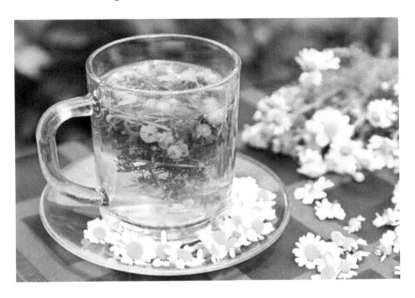

Chamomile is an herb traditionally used to reduce muscle tension, soothe digestion, and reduce anxiety, which may help induce sleep.

Sip a cup of hot chamomile tea after dinner. But don't drink it too close to the bed or you may have to get up in the middle of the night to go to the bathroom.

4. Lavender Flower

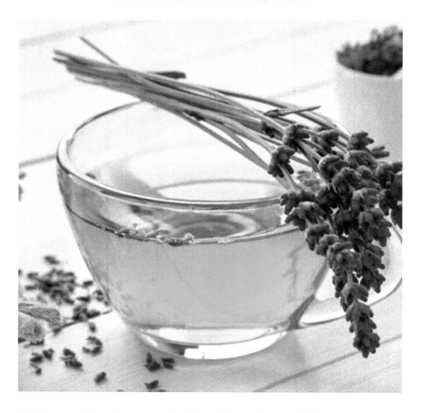

The lavender plant can be found on almost all continents. It produces purple flowers that, when dried, have a variety of household uses.

Moreover, lavender's soothing fragrance is believed to enhance sleep.

In fact, several studies show that simply smelling lavender oil shortly before sleep may be enough to improve sleep quality. This effect appears particularly strong in those with mild insomnia, especially females and young individuals.

5. Passionflower

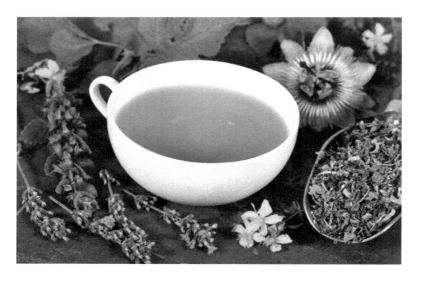

Passionflower, also known as Passiflora incarnata or maypop, is a popular herbal remedy for insomnia.

The species of passionflower linked to sleep improvements are native to North America. They're also currently cultivated in Europe, Asia, Africa, and Australia.

Passionflower's sleep-promoting effects have been demonstrated in animal studies.

6. Ginkgo Biloba

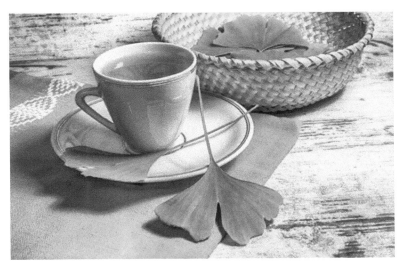

According to older studies, consuming around 240 mg of this natural herb 30–60 minutes before bed may help reduce stress, enhance relaxation, and promote sleep. Animal studies are also promising. Ginkgo Biloba very good to reduce insomnia naturally.

7. Kava

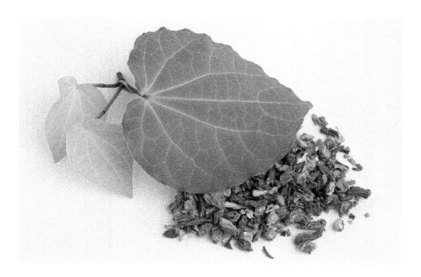

Kava also known as kava kava, is an herbal remedy that's used for stress and anxiety relief and insomnia. Kava acts by way of a different mechanism.

Some say that it may induce relaxation without hindering memory or motor function.

8. Acupuncture

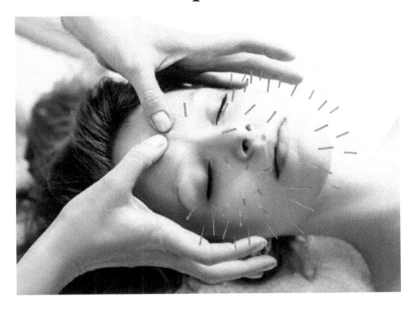

Acupuncture is often used in traditional Chinese medicine for the treatment of insomnia. This procedure involves the insertion of very fine needles.

Sometimes in combination with electrical stimulus or with heat produced by burning specific herbs) into the skin at specific acupuncture points in order to influence the functioning of the body.

The results of recent studies have shown acupuncture improved sleep quality in people with insomnia.

9. Yoga

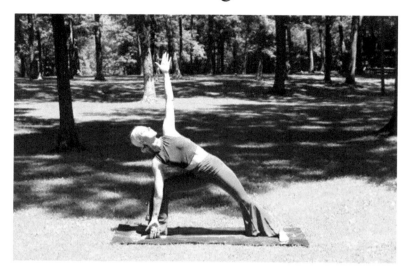

We're all told we should get more sleep. If you live with insomnia, however, the idea of sleeping soundly through the night may seem like a dream.

You've probably already tried counting sheep backward and forward, so your next step may be to add a gentle yoga practice to your nightly routine.

A Harvard Medical Source study found that a regular yoga practice improved sleep efficiency, total sleep time, and how quickly participants fell asleep, among other improvements for those living with insomnia.

Though it may be tempting to think you should tire yourself out with intense workouts before bed, you actually want to calm your nervous system and wind down from your day. The key to yoga for sleep is to go for calm and restorative poses.

10. Pomegranate Fruit

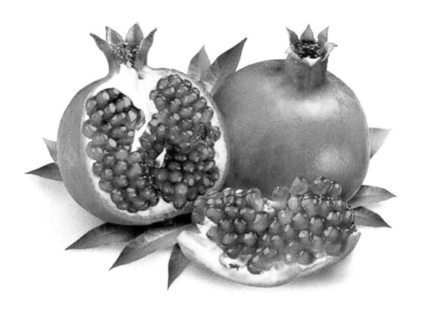

Pomegranate, commonly referred as "Divine Fruit" is used in ayurveda to maintain a balanced level of body temperature. It has lot of nutrients like vitamin c, potassium and antioxidants.

Due to its antibacterial and antiviral properties, it can be used to prevent many infectious diseases. Pomegranate has enriched vitamin c nutrients which is the key for optimal sleep. Consuming more amount of pomegranate promotes healthy sleep patterns and helps you to sleep effortlessly.

11. Almonds

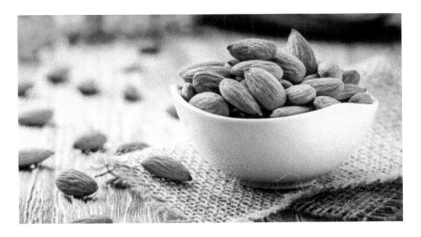

Best food to eat before sleep. Almonds contain sleep-supporting amino acid tryptophan, as well as the nutrient magnesium, as a natural muscle relaxer.

Protein in almonds will keep you full all night and help to regulate your sleep cycle.

12. Hot Milk

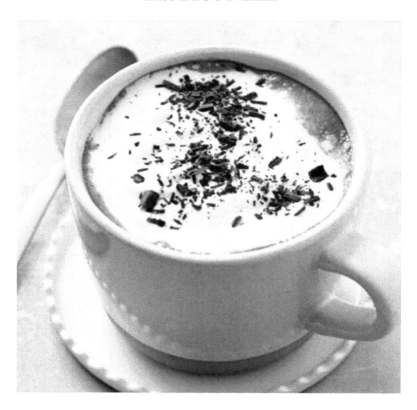

Milk is the rich source of amino acid tryptophan which has a calming effect on the body that helps to control melatonin production.

Milk is also a great source of calcium, a mineral that plays a role in the regulation of melatonin in the body.

13. Cherries

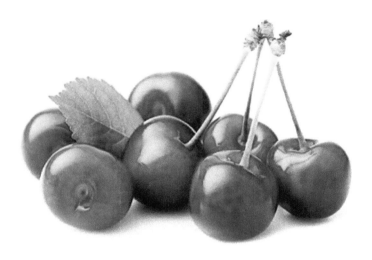

Cherries are also high in melatonin, which helps to regulate the sleep cycle. Experts and research indicate you should eat cherries or cherry drink before going to bed to fight with sleeplessness.

14. Corns

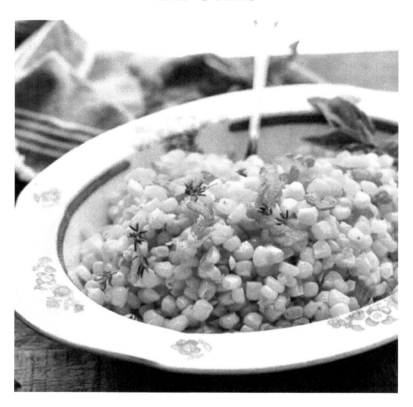

Due to a high amount of carbs, corns can easily regulate the sleep cycle. Carbs stimulate insulin which indirectly makes tryptophan.

Higher-glycemic carbs are more effective than lower-glycemic carbs, but sugary carbs are not good for blood sugar causes sleeplessness.

15. Spinach

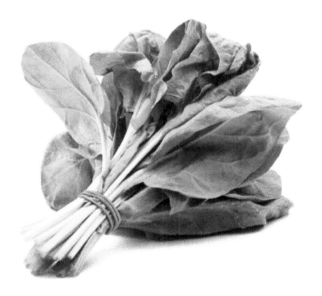

Another sleep boosting food is spinach which is high in magnesium that naturally relaxes the tiring muscles, calming the body and regulate the sleep cycle.

Magnesiumin spinch help prevent leg cramps. Good source of calcium which helps the brain use tryptophan to manufacture meatonin, a sleep enhancing hormone.

16. Lettuce

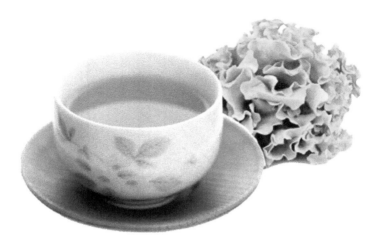

Lettuce contains an opium-related compound which is known to promote healthy sleep. If you're having difficulty sleeping, make lettuce a regular item on your evening menu.

17. Banana

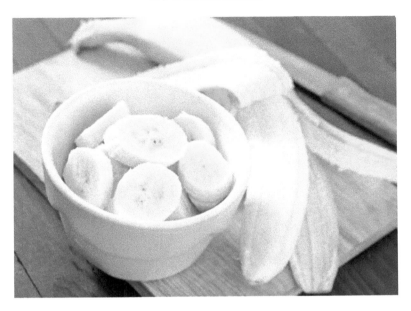

Bananas help fight insomnia in three powerful ways." They are a source of magnesium, serotonin, and melatonin," both precursors to melatonin and serotonin, important hormones that regulate sleep says Palinski-Wade.

"Serotonin is a neurotransmitter that helps to regulate sleep as well as mood and appetite and magnesium promotes sleep by helping to decrease the level of cortisol in the body, a hormone that is known to interrupt sleep."

18. Basil

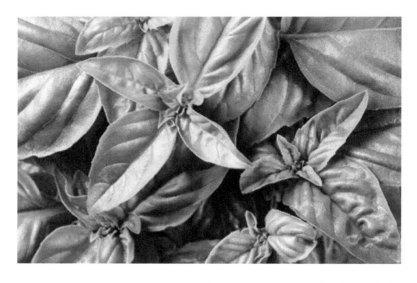

"This plant actually contains sedative properties, which can help you fall asleep and stay asleep. And as a bonus, it not only helps promote sleep, but can help reduce indigestion," says Palinski-Wade, which is itself a major sleep-interrupter.

"Research on this shows the sedative properties come mostly from the hydroalcoholic extract and essential oil of O. basilicum (basil). So we possibly can say incorporating essential oil from basil seeds would be a good way to gain these benefits.

There are liquid basil extracts available on the market that can be used to flavor food, as a supplement, or as an essential oil,"

19. Kiwi

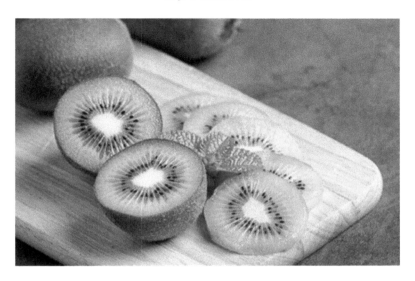

The kiwi or kiwifruit is a small, oval-shaped fruit popularly associated with New Zealand even though it is grown in numerous countries. There are both green and gold varieties, but green kiwis are produced in greater numbers.

Kiwifruit possess numerous vitamins and minerals, most notably vitamins C and E as well as potassium and folate.

Some research has found that eating kiwi can improve sleep. In a study, people who ate two kiwis one hour before bedtime found that they fell asleep faster, slept more, and had better sleep quality.

It is not known for sure why kiwis may help with sleep, but researchers believe that it could relate to their antioxidant properties, ability to address folate deficiencies, and/or high concentration of serotonin.

20. Fatty Fish

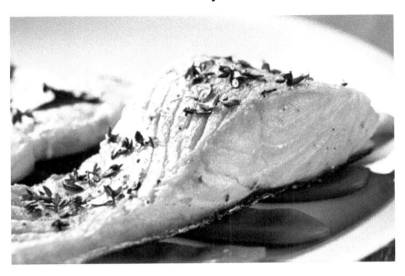

A research study found that fatty fish may be a good food for better sleep. The study over a period of months found that people who ate salmon three times per week had better overall sleep as well as improved daytime functioning.

Researchers believe that fatty fish may help sleep by providing a healthy dose of vitamin D and omega-3 fatty acids, which are involved in the body's regulation of serotonin.

This study focused particularly on fish consumption during winter months when vitamin D levels tend to be lower.

21. Walnuts

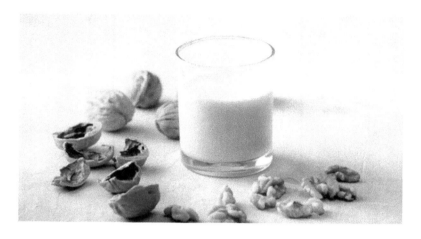

Walnuts are a popular type of tree nut. They're abundant in many nutrients, providing over 19 vitamins and minerals, in addition to 1.9 grams of fiber, in a 1-ounce (28-gram) serving. Walnuts are particularly rich in magnesium, phosphorus, manganese, and copper.

Additionally, walnuts are a great source of healthy fats, including omega-3 fatty acids and linoleic acid. They also provide 4.3 grams of protein per ounce, which may be beneficial for reducing appetite.

Walnuts may also boost heart health. They've been studied for their ability to reduce high cholesterol levels, which are a major risk factor for heart disease

What's more, some researchers claim that eating walnuts improves sleep quality, as they're one of the best food sources of melatonin.

The fatty acid makeup of walnuts may also contribute to better sleep. They provide alpha-linolenic acid (ALA), an omega-3 fatty acid that's converted to DHA in the body. DHA may increase serotonin production.

22. Watermelons

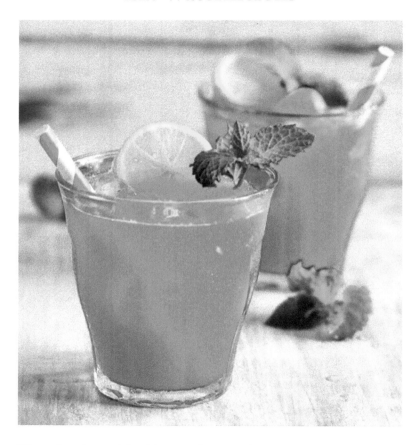

These bright and highly enriching melons are indeed a blessing in disguise. A cup of diced watermelon pieces just before bedtime helps you to stay hydrated throughout the night and helps to keep post-dinner hunger pangs at bay, thanks to its higher fibre content and volume.

Therefore, since you are adequately hydrated before sleeping, the body doesn't urge you in the middle of the night to fulfil its thirst requirements, and you land up sleeping peacefully.

However, make it a point to consume these melons in moderation because they may wake you up in the middle of the night to make a quick trip to the washroom thanks to their high-water content.

23. Pistachios

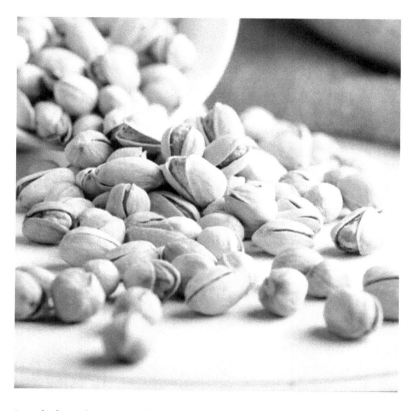

Loaded with essential nutrients such as vitamin B6, proteins, magnesium, pistachios can help induce sleep.

But again, consume them in moderation because anything that is high in calories can make you stay awake rather than inducing sleep.

24. White Rice

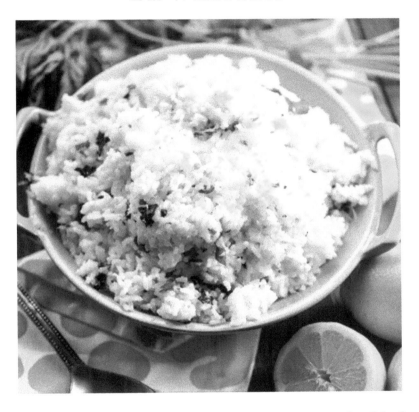

Many amongst us have experienced this! Consume a plateful of white rice for lunch, and you are bound to feel sleepy and lazy.

White rice is high in carbohydrates and low in fibre. It also has a high glycemic index — which is a measure of how quickly a food item increases your blood sugar.

Studies show that when food items with a high glycemic index are consumed a few hours before bedtime, they may help in improving sleep quality.

25. Prunes

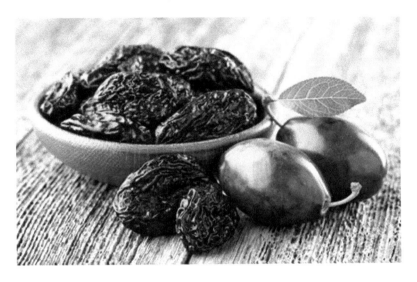

Like walnuts, prunes also aid in promoting the levels of the sleep hormone Melatonin. Along with helping you sleep, prunes also up your calcium, magnesium, and vitamin B6 levels.

26. Barley Grass Powder

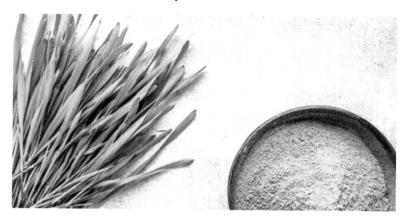

Barley grass powder is rich in several sleep-promoting compounds, including GABA, calcium, tryptophan, zinc, potassium, and magnesium.

According to a 2018 research review, barley grass powder may promote sleep and help prevent a range of other conditions.

People can mix barley grass powder into smoothies, scrambled eggs, salad dressings, and soups. It is available in some food stores and online.

27. Grapefruit

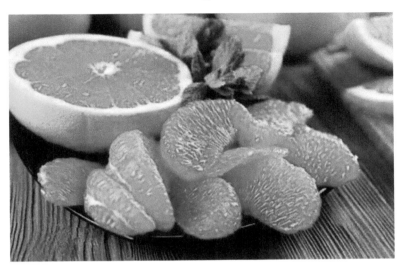

It is a proven fact that lycopene, an antioxidant, improves the way of sleeping a lot. Grape fruit is one of the good sources of lycopene which promotes a healthy sleep cycle. Drinking a glass of grape fruit juice before going to bed helps you to get better sleep without tossing and turning around.

It also contain tryptophan, a chemical which secretes after a big meal that makes you sleepy. Hence, grape fruits can regulate the sleep cycles way a lot better. It has absolutely no side effects as the minerals from grapefruit are easily soluble in water which can be easily flushed out from the body.

28. Pinneaple

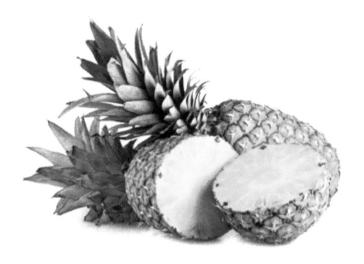

Pineapple is used widely to treat digestive and inflammation problems. So, how come it will help you to get good sleep? It has abundant source of melatonin which increases the serum levels, especially for males.

The digestive enzyme named bromelain in pineapple helps to relieve stiffness, muscle pains and also reduces inflammations. Hence it soothes the body pain and provides a natural way to sleep better.

It acts as a great medicine for fibromyalgia and other musculoskeletal pains which are the major causes for problematic sleep cycles.

29. Orange

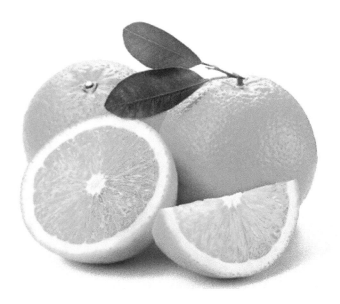

Oranges are considered to be the world's healthiest food. The great source calcium and vitamin B in oranges produces melatonin efficiently and relaxes your body quickly. Hence, it can be used effectively to treat any kind of sleep related problems.

An orange can fulfill up to 72% of daily requirement of vitamin C. It can also be used effectively to treat constipation, hair loss, rheumatic arthritis and diabetes etc.You can even try blood oranges in early spring season, since it has richer antioxidant content.

30. Strawberry

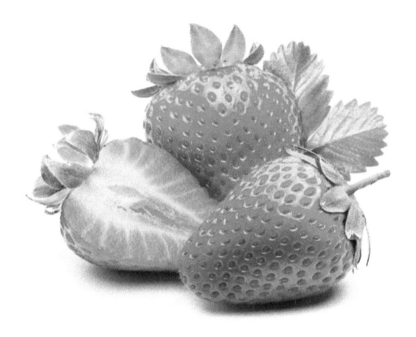

Strawberry is not only a popular artificial flavor, but also a good sleep inducer. Strawberry is packed with many nutrients like vitamin c, calcium, folate, potassium, manganese and dietary fibre.

You can snack on a bowl of strawberry before bed which boost up the sleep regulating melatonin that paves way to have a good sleep.

31. Taichi

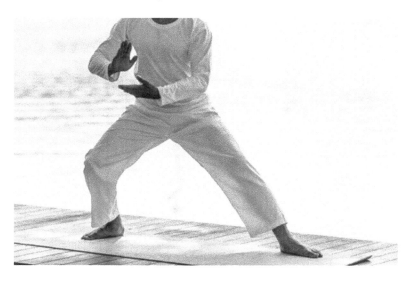

Tai Chi significantly improved sleep quality in both healthy adults and patients with chronic health conditions, which suggests that Tai Chi may be considered as an alternative behavioral therapy in the treatment of insomnia.

Tai Chi originated in China as a martial art, focusing on the mind and body as an interconnected system, on breathing, and on keeping a calm state of mind with a goal toward deep states of relaxation.

32. Raw Honey

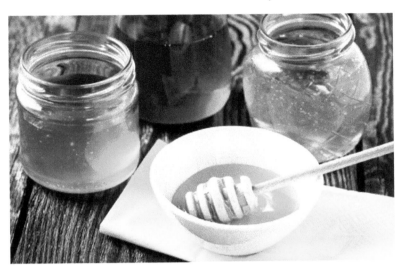

While most folks keep honey in the pantry, you may want to grab a bottle for your nightstand, too. Raw and unfiltered local honey can hydrate your skin, soothe your throat, help heal wounds and sweeten everything it touches, but it can also help you get a sweet night's sleep. Raw honey, eaten just before bed, helps you snooze in two general ways:

#a) It provides easy-to-access fuel for your brain throughout the night. Specifically, it restocks your liver's glycogen. Low levels of glycogen tell your brain that it's time to eat. If you haven't eaten in several hours when you go to sleep, this "hunger" can cause you to wake up in the middle of the night and sleep less soundly.

#b) Honey helps your brain release melatonin, the hormone that your body uses to restore itself during sleep. This happens through a series of transformations in your brain: honey's sugars spike your insulin levels, releasing tryptophan, which becomes serotonin, which becomes melatonin.

Author Bio

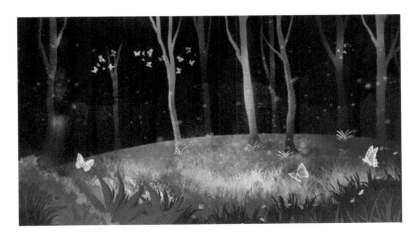

Allah SWT (God) Say:

"And of his signs is your sleep by day and by night and your seeking of his great bounty. Indeed, in that are signs for those who listen"

(from The Noble Quran Surah Ar-Rum)

And it is He who sends down rain from the sky, and We produce thereby the growth of all things. We produce from it greenery from which We produce grains arranged in layers. And from the palm trees, of its emerging fruit are clusters hanging low. And [We produce] gardens of grapevines and olives and pomegranates, similar yet varied. Look at [each of] its fruit when it yields and [at] its ripening. Indeed in that are signs for a people who believe.

(from The Noble Quran Surah An-Naml)

43

References

Kierlin L (November 2008). "Sleeping without a pill: nonpharmacologic treatments for insomnia". Journal of Psychiatric Practice.

Attarian HP (2003). Clinical Handbook of Insomnia. Springer Science & Business Media.

PhD, Jack D. Edinger (2013). Insomnia, An Issue of Sleep Medicine Clinics. Elsevier Health Sciences.

"What causes insomnia?". National Heart, Lung, and Blood Institute. 3 July 2013.

Lee-chiong T (24 April 2008). Sleep Medicine: Essentials and Review. Oxford University Press.

Lader M, Cardinali DP, Pandi-Perumal SR (2006). Sleep and sleep disorders: a neuropsychopharmacological approach. Georgetown, Tex.: Landes Bioscience

Lightning Source UK Ltd.
Milton Keynes UK
UKHW020804180621
385732UK00001B/183